CANCER- FIGHTING KITCHEN

30+ Delectable Plant-Based Anticancer Recipes revealing the secrets to combat the Disease using natural therapies.

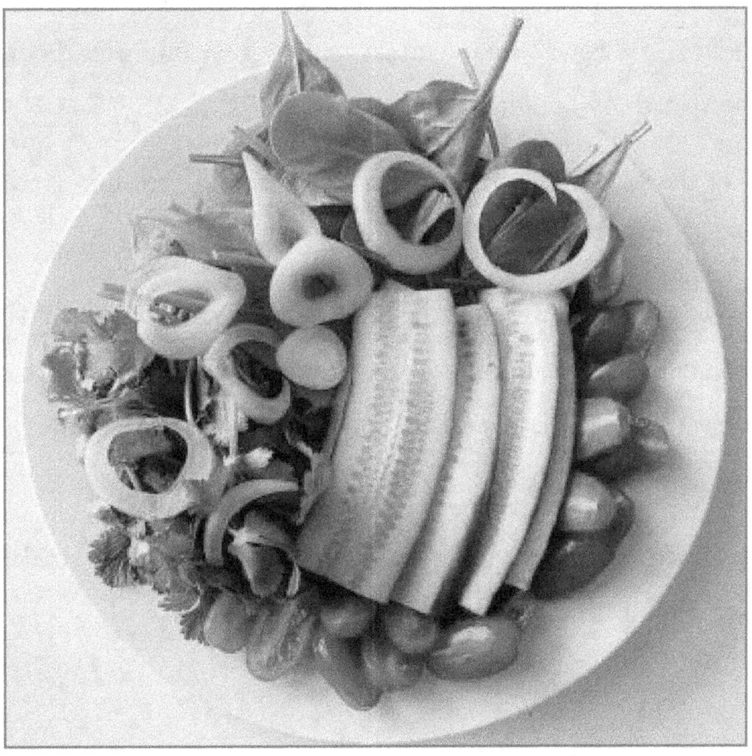

SHARON OT WASHINGTON

Disclaimer: Any medical or nutritional information presented in this book is intended for informational purposes only and should not be considered as a substitute for professional advice.

Consult with your healthcare professional before making significant dietary changes.

TABLE OF CONTENTS

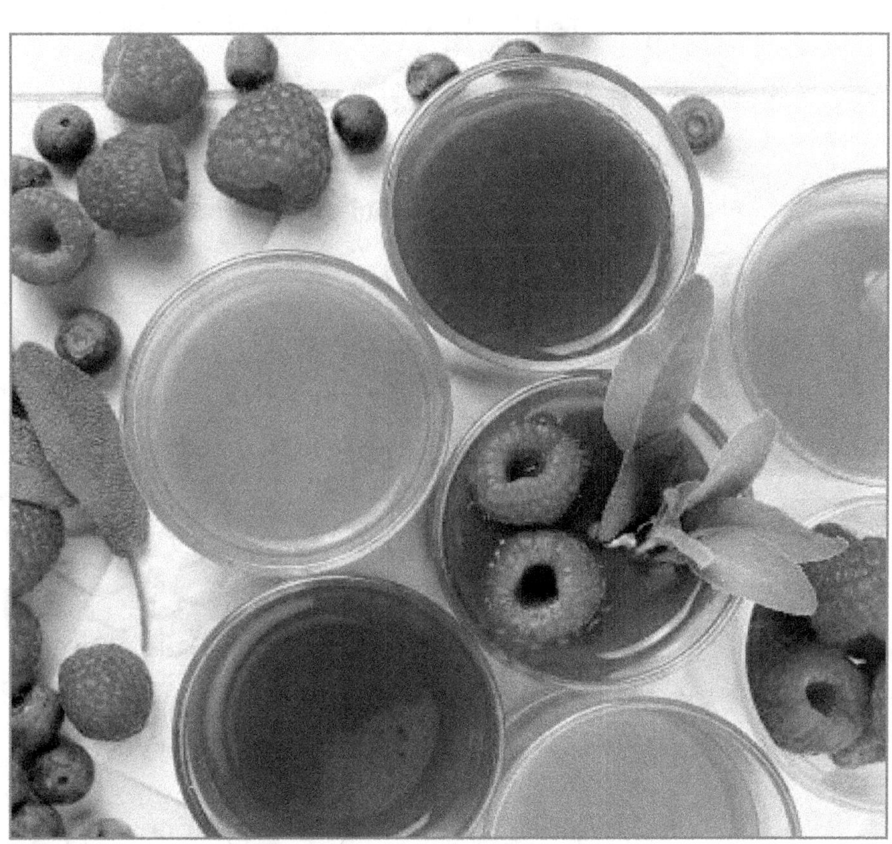

INTRODUCTION

Embark on a transformative culinary journey with our exclusive collection of 42 plant-based, anticancer recipes meticulously crafted to empower your health and vitality.

In our "Cancer-Fighting Kitchen," discover the intersection of exquisite flavors and natural therapies as we unveil the secrets to combat disease through the art of nourishing cuisine.

Each recipe serves as a gastronomic revelation, showcasing the harmonious fusion of nutrient-packed ingredients designed to fortify your body's defenses.

From the invigorating "Lemon Herb Baked Tofu" to the heartwarming "Pumpkin and Turmeric Soup," these dishes not only tantalize the taste buds but also embody the principles of a wholesome, plant-powered lifestyle.

Delve into the vibrant hues and robust aromas of our creations, where each carefully curated ingredient plays a vital role in promoting wellness. Our aim is to redefine your relationship with food, offering a symphony of flavors that not only satiates but also serves as a celebration of life and health. Welcome to a world where deliciousness meets disease prevention — a world where each bite becomes a step towards a resilient and thriving you.

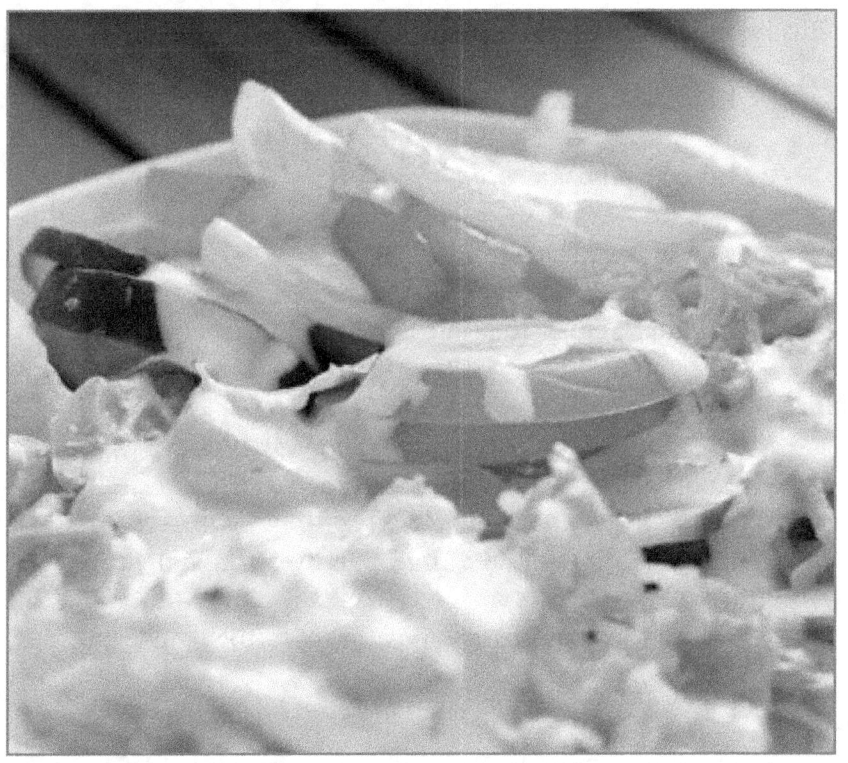

Recipe 1: Quinoa Power Bowl

Ingredients:

*   1 cup quinoa

*   2 cups broccoli florets

*   1 cup cherry tomatoes, halved

*   1 cup carrots, julienned

*   1 cup kale, chopped

*   1/4 cup pumpkin seeds

*   1/4 cup extra-virgin olive oil

*   Salt and pepper to taste

Instructions:

1.   Cook quinoa according to package instructions.

2.   Heat the olive oil in a large pan over medium heat.

3.   Add broccoli, cherry tomatoes, carrots, and kale. Sauté until the vegetables are tender.

4.   Combine cooked quinoa with sautéed vegetables in a bowl.

5.   Sprinkle pumpkin seeds on top.

6.   Season with salt and pepper, to taste.

Nutritional Value (per serving):

*   Calories: 400

*   Protein: 15g

*   Carbohydrates: 55g

*   Fiber: 10g

*   Fat: 18g

Recipe 2: Turmeric-Infused Lentil Soup

Ingredients:

*   1 cup red lentils

*   1 onion, diced

*   3 cloves garlic, minced

*   1 tablespoon fresh ginger, grated

*   1 teaspoon turmeric powder

- • 4 cups vegetable broth

- • 1 can (14 oz) diced tomatoes

- • 2 cups spinach, chopped

- • Salt and pepper to taste

Instructions:

1. Rinse the lentils under cold water.

2. In a large pot, sauté onions, garlic, and ginger until fragrant.

3. Add turmeric powder and stir.

4. Pour in vegetable broth, lentils, and diced tomatoes.

5. Simmer for 20 minutes or until the lentils are tender.

6. Cook until the spinach is wilted, stirring often.

7. Season with salt and pepper, to taste.

Nutritional Value (per serving):

- • Calories: 320

- • Protein: 18g

- • Carbohydrates: 45g

- Fiber: 12g

- Fat: 6g

Recipe 3: Berry Blast Smoothie Bowl

Ingredients:

- 1 cup of mixed berries (blueberries, raspberries and strawberries)

- 1 banana, frozen

- 1/2 cup almond milk

- 2 tablespoons chia seeds

- 1 tablespoon almond butter

- Granola and sliced almonds for topping

Instructions:

1. Blend mixed berries, frozen banana, almond milk, chia seeds, and almond butter until smooth.

2. Pour the smoothie into a bowl.

3.   Top with granola and sliced almonds.

Nutritional Value (per serving):

*   Calories: 280

*   Protein: 8g

*   Carbohydrates: 40g

*   Fiber: 10g

*   Fat: 10g

Recipe 4: Avocado & Chickpea Salad

Ingredients:

*   2 cups canned chickpeas, drained and rinsed

*   1 avocado, diced

*   1 cucumber, diced

*   1 cup cherry tomatoes, halved

*   1/4 cup red onion, finely chopped

- Fresh cilantro, chopped

- Juice of 1 lemon

- 2 tablespoons extra-virgin olive oil

- Salt and pepper to taste

Instructions:

1. In a large bowl, combine chickpeas, avocado, cucumber, cherry tomatoes, red onion, and cilantro.

2. Drizzle olive oil and lemon juice over the salad.

3. Gently toss to combine all the ingredients.

4. Season with salt and pepper, to taste.

Nutritional Value (per serving):

- Calories: 320

- Protein: 12g

- Carbohydrates: 38g

- Fiber: 12g

- Fat: 16g

Recipe 5: Green Tea-Infused Quinoa Salad

Ingredients:

* 1 cup quinoa, cooked and cooled

* 1 cup edamame, shelled

* 1 bell pepper, diced

* 1 cup cucumber, sliced

* 2 green onions, thinly sliced

* 1/4 cup fresh parsley, chopped

* 2 tablespoons sesame oil

* 2 tablespoons rice vinegar

* 1 tablespoon soy sauce

* 1 teaspoon honey

Instructions:

1.   In a large bowl, combine quinoa, edamame, bell pepper, cucumber, green onions, and parsley.

2.	In a small bowl, whisk together sesame oil, rice vinegar, soy sauce, and honey.

3.	Pour the dressing over the salad and toss until well coated.

4.	Allow at least 30 minutes before serving to chill.

Nutritional Value (per serving):

- Calories: 280

- Protein: 14g

- Carbohydrates: 32g

- Fiber: 6g

- Fat: 12g

Recipe 6: Rainbow Stuffed Bell Peppers

Ingredients:

- 4 bell peppers, halved

- 1 cup quinoa, cooked

- 1 can (15 oz) black beans, washed and drained

- 1 cup corn kernels

- 1 cup cherry tomatoes, diced

- 1/2 cup red onion, finely chopped

- 1/4 cup fresh cilantro, chopped

- 1 teaspoon cumin

- Juice of 2 limes

- Salt and pepper to taste

Instructions:

1.   Preheat the oven to 375°F (190°C).

2.   In a large bowl, mix quinoa, black beans, corn, cherry tomatoes, red onion, cilantro, cumin, lime juice, salt, and pepper.

3.   Fill each bell pepper half halfway with the quinoa mixture.

4.   Place stuffed peppers in a baking dish and bake for 25-30 minutes until peppers are tender.

Nutritional Value (per serving):

- Calories: 320

- Protein: 14g

- Carbohydrates: 60g

- Fiber: 12g

- Fat: 5g

Recipe 7: Broccoli and Almond Stir-Fry

Ingredients:

- 2 cups broccoli florets

- 1 cup snap peas, trimmed

- 1 carrot, julienned

- 1 bell pepper, sliced

- 1 cup tofu, cubed

- 2 tablespoons sesame oil

- 3 tablespoons low-sodium soy sauce

- 2 tablespoons rice vinegar

- 1 tablespoon maple syrup

- 1/4 cup almonds, sliced

- Brown rice (optional, for serving)

Instructions:

1. In a wok or large skillet, heat sesame oil over medium-high heat.

2. Add the tofu and stir-fry until golden brown. Remove the tofu from the pan and set it aside.

3. In the same pan, stir-fry broccoli, snap peas, carrots, and bell peppers until vegetables are tender-crisp.

4. In a small bowl, whisk together soy sauce, rice vinegar, and maple syrup. Pour over the vegetables.

5. Add the cooked tofu back to the pan and toss until everything is well coated.

6. Serve over brown rice and garnish with sliced almonds.

Nutritional Value (per serving):

- Calories: 380

- Protein: 18g

- Carbohydrates: 35g

- Fiber: 9g

- Fat: 20g

Recipe 8: Spinach and Walnut Pesto Pasta

Ingredients:

- 8 oz. whole grain or gluten-free pasta

- 2 cups fresh spinach

- 1/2 cup walnuts

- 2 cloves garlic

- 1/2 cup nutritional yeast

- Juice of 1 lemon

- 1/4 cup extra-virgin olive oil

- Salt and pepper to taste

Instructions:

1. Cook pasta according to package instructions.

2. In a food processor, combine spinach, walnuts, garlic, nutritional yeast, and lemon juice.

3. Pulse until the ingredients are finely chopped.

4. With the food processor running, slowly pour in the olive oil until the pesto is well combined.

5. Toss the cooked pasta with the spinach and walnut pesto.

6. Season with salt and pepper, to taste.

Nutritional Value (per serving):

- Calories: 420

- Protein: 15g

- Carbohydrates: 50g

- Fiber: 8g

- Fat: 20g

Recipe 9: Berry Quinoa Parfait

Ingredients:

- 1 cup cooked quinoa, cooled

- 1 cup mixed berries (strawberries, blueberries, raspberries)

- 1/2 cup coconut yogurt

- 1 tablespoon chia seeds

- 2 tablespoons honey or maple syrup

- 1/4 cup sliced almonds

Instructions:

1. In a glass or bowl, layer cooked quinoa, mixed berries, and coconut yogurt.

2. Sprinkle chia seeds on top.

3. Drizzle with honey or maple syrup.

4. Garnish with sliced almonds.

5. Repeat for additional layers if desired.

Nutritional Value (per serving):

- Calories: 350

- Protein: 10g

- Carbohydrates: 45g

- Fiber: 8g

- Fat: 15g

Recipe 10: Sweet Potato and Kale Buddha Bowl

Ingredients:

- 2 medium sweet potatoes, cubed

- 2 cups kale, stems removed and chopped

- 1 cup chickpeas, cooked

- 1 avocado, sliced

- 2 tablespoons tahini

- Juice of 1 lime

- 1 tablespoon olive oil

- Salt and pepper to taste

Instructions:

1. Preheat the oven to 400°F (200°C).

2. Toss sweet potato cubes with olive oil, salt, and pepper. Roast for 25–30 minutes until golden.

3. In a large bowl, massage kale with lime juice until slightly wilted.

4. Assemble bowls with roasted sweet potatoes, massaged kale, chickpeas, and avocado slices.

5. Drizzle with tahini and season with additional salt and pepper if desired.

Nutritional Value (per serving):

- Calories: 380

- Protein: 12g

- Carbohydrates: 45g

- Fiber: 14g

- Fat: 18g

Recipe 11: Mango and Black Bean Salad

Ingredients:

- 1 can (15 oz) black beans, drained and rinsed

- 2 mangoes, diced

- 1 red bell pepper, diced

- 1/2 red onion, finely chopped

- 1 jalapeño, seeded and minced

- 1/4 cup fresh cilantro, chopped

- Juice of 2 limes

- 2 tablespoons olive oil

- Salt and pepper to taste

Instructions:

1. In a large bowl, combine black beans, diced mangoes, red bell pepper, red onion, jalapeño, and cilantro.

2. In a small bowl, whisk together the lime juice and olive oil. Pour over the salad.

3. Toss the salad until well combined.

4. Season with salt and pepper, to taste.

Nutritional Value (per serving):

- Calories: 320

- Protein: 9g

- Carbohydrates: 55g

- Fiber: 14g

- Fat: 10g

Recipe 12: Lentil and Vegetable Curry

Ingredients:

- 1 cup dried green lentils

- 1 onion, diced

- 3 cloves garlic, minced

- 1 tablespoon ginger, grated

- 2 carrots, sliced

- 1 zucchini, diced

- 1 can (14 oz) diced tomatoes

- 1 can (14 oz) coconut milk

- 2 tablespoons curry powder

- 1 teaspoon turmeric

- Salt and pepper to taste

Instructions:

1. Cook lentils according to package instructions.

2. In a large pot, sauté onion, garlic, and ginger until fragrant.

3. Add carrots, zucchini, diced tomatoes, coconut milk, curry powder, turmeric, salt, and pepper.

4. Simmer for 20 minutes until the vegetables are tender.

5. Stir in the cooked lentils and cook for an additional 10 minutes.

Nutritional Value (per serving):

- Calories: 380

- Protein: 15g

- Carbohydrates: 45g

- Fiber: 12g

- Fat: 18g

Recipe 13: Cauliflower and Chickpea Tacos

Ingredients:

- 1 head cauliflower, cut into florets

- 1 can (15 oz) chickpeas, drained and rinsed

- 1 tablespoon taco seasoning

- 8 small whole-grain or corn tortillas

- 1 cup shredded purple cabbage

- 1 avocado, sliced

- 1/4 cup fresh cilantro, chopped

- Lime wedges for serving

Instructions:

1. Preheat the oven to 400°F (200°C).

2. Toss cauliflower florets and chickpeas with taco seasoning.

3. Roast in the oven for 20–25 minutes until cauliflower is golden and chickpeas are crispy.

4. Warm tortillas in a dry skillet.

5. Assemble tacos with roasted cauliflower and chickpeas, shredded cabbage, avocado slices, and cilantro.

6. Serve with lime wedges.

Nutritional Value (per serving):

- Calories: 320

- Protein: 10g

- Carbohydrates: 45g

- Fiber: 12g

- Fat: 14g

Recipe 14: Almond-Crusted Baked Eggplant

Ingredients:

- 1 large eggplant, sliced into rounds

- 1 cup almond meal

- 1 teaspoon smoked paprika

- 1/2 teaspoon garlic powder

- 2 flax eggs (2 tablespoons ground flaxseed + 6 tablespoons water)

- Salt and pepper to taste

- Marinara sauce for dipping

Instructions:

1. Preheat the oven to 375°F (190°C).

2. In a shallow bowl, mix almond meal, smoked paprika, garlic powder, salt, and pepper.

3. Dip eggplant slices in flax eggs, then coat with the almond mixture.

4. Place them on a baking sheet lined with parchment paper.

5. Bake for 25–30 minutes until the coating is golden and crispy.

6. Serve with marinara sauce for dipping.

Nutritional Value (per serving):

- Calories: 250

- Protein: 8g

- Carbohydrates: 30g

- Fiber: 10g

- Fat: 12g

Recipe 15: Mediterranean Quinoa Salad

Ingredients:

- 1 cup quinoa, cooked and cooled

- 1 cucumber, diced

- 1 cup cherry tomatoes, halved

- 1/2 cup Kalamata olives, sliced

- 1/4 cup red onion, finely chopped

- 1/2 cup crumbled feta cheese (optional)

- Juice of 1 lemon

- 3 tablespoons extra-virgin olive oil

- Fresh oregano, chopped

- Salt and pepper to taste

Instructions:

1. In a large bowl, combine quinoa, cucumber, cherry tomatoes, olives, red onion, and feta cheese.

2. In a small bowl, whisk together the lemon juice, olive oil, oregano, salt, and pepper.

3. Pour the dressing over the salad and toss until well combined.

4. Chill in the refrigerator for at least 30 minutes before serving.

Nutritional Value (per serving):

- Calories: 300

- Protein: 10g

- Carbohydrates: 35g

- Fiber: 7g

- Fat: 15g

Recipe 16: Teriyaki Tofu Stir-Fry

Ingredients:

- 1 block extra-firm tofu, pressed and cubed

- 2 cups broccoli florets

- 1 bell pepper, sliced

- 1 carrot, julienned

- 1 cup snow peas, trimmed

- 1/4 cup low-sodium teriyaki sauce

- 2 tablespoons sesame oil

- 2 tablespoons sesame seeds

- Green onions for garnish

Instructions:

1. In a wok or large skillet, heat sesame oil over medium-high heat.

2. Add the tofu cubes and cook until golden brown.

3. Add broccoli, bell pepper, carrot, and snow peas. Stir-fry until vegetables are tender-crisp.

4. Pour teriyaki sauce over the tofu and vegetables, tossing to coat.

5. Sprinkle sesame seeds and garnish with green onions.

6. Serve over brown rice or quinoa, if desired.

Nutritional Value (per serving):

- Calories: 350

- Protein: 18g

- Carbohydrates: 30g

- Fiber: 8g

- Fat: 18g

Recipe 17: Chia Seed Pudding Parfait

Ingredients:

- 1/4 cup chia seeds

- 1 cup almond milk

- 1 teaspoon vanilla extract

- 1 tablespoon maple syrup

- 1 cup mixed berries (raspberries, strawberries and blueberries,)

- 1/4 cup granola

- Fresh mint for garnish

Instructions:

1. In a jar, mix chia seeds, almond milk, vanilla extract, and maple syrup. Stir well and refrigerate overnight.

2. In the morning, stir the chia pudding to ensure it's well set.

3. In serving glasses, layer chia pudding, mixed berries, and granola.

4. Repeat for additional layers if desired.

5. Garnish with fresh mint before serving.

Nutritional Value (per serving):

- Calories: 280

- Protein: 8g

- Carbohydrates: 35g

- Fiber: 10g

- Fat: 12g

Recipe 18: Roasted Brussels sprouts and Pomegranate Salad

Ingredients:

- 1 lb. Brussels sprouts, halved

- 1 tablespoon olive oil

- Salt and pepper to taste

- 1/2 cup pomegranate seeds

- 1/4 cup chopped pecans

- 1 tablespoon balsamic glaze

Instructions:

1. Preheat the oven to 400°F (200°C).

2. Toss Brussels sprouts with olive oil, salt, and pepper.

3. Roast for 20–25 minutes until Brussels sprouts are golden and crispy.

4. In a serving bowl, combine roasted Brussels sprouts, pomegranate seeds, and chopped pecans.

5. Drizzle with a balsamic glaze before serving.

Nutritional Value (per serving):

- Calories: 180

- Protein: 5g

- Carbohydrates: 25g

- Fiber: 8g

- Fat: 10g

Recipe 19: Lemon Herb Baked Tofu

Ingredients:

- 1 block extra-firm tofu, pressed and sliced

- Juice of 2 lemons

- Zest of 1 lemon

- 2 tablespoons olive oil

- 1 tablespoon fresh thyme, chopped

- 1 tablespoon fresh rosemary, chopped

- 2 cloves garlic, minced

- Salt and pepper to taste

Instructions:

1. Preheat the oven to 375°F (190°C).

2. In a bowl, whisk together lemon juice, lemon zest, olive oil, thyme, rosemary, garlic, salt, and pepper.

3. Place tofu slices in a baking dish and pour the lemon herb marinade over them.

4. Bake for 25–30 minutes until the tofu is golden and infused with flavors.

Nutritional Value (per serving):

- Calories: 240

- Protein: 12g

- Carbohydrates: 8g

- Fiber: 3g

- Fat: 18g

Recipe 20: Pumpkin and Turmeric Soup

Ingredients:

- 1 can (15 oz) pumpkin puree

- 1 onion, diced

- 2 carrots, chopped

- 1 apple, peeled and diced

- 1 teaspoon turmeric powder

- 1/2 teaspoon cinnamon

- 4 cups vegetable broth

- 1 cup coconut milk

- Salt and pepper to taste

- Pumpkin seeds for garnish

Instructions:

1. In a pot, sauté the onion, carrots, and apple until softened.

2. Add the turmeric and cinnamon, stirring to coat the vegetables.

3. Pour in vegetable broth and bring to a simmer.

4. Stir in the pumpkin puree and coconut milk.

5. Simmer for 15-20 minutes.

6. Blend the soup until smooth using an immersion blender.

7. Season with salt and pepper, and garnish with pumpkin seeds before serving.

Nutritional Value (per serving):

- Calories: 220

- Protein: 3g

- Carbohydrates: 30g

- Fiber: 8g

- Fat: 10g

Recipe 21: Grilled Portobello Mushrooms with Herbed Quinoa

Ingredients:

- 4 large Portobello mushrooms, stems removed

- 1 cup quinoa, cooked

- 1/4 cup fresh parsley, chopped

- 2 tablespoons fresh basil, chopped

- 2 tablespoons balsamic vinegar

- 2 tablespoons olive oil

- Salt and pepper to taste

Instructions:

1. Preheat the grill to medium-high heat.

2. In a bowl, mix cooked quinoa with parsley, basil, balsamic vinegar, olive oil, salt, and pepper.

3. Grill Portobello mushrooms for 5–7 minutes per side.

4. Spoon herbed quinoa onto the mushrooms before serving.

Nutritional Value (per serving):

- Calories: 280

- Protein: 10g

- Carbohydrates: 35g

- Fiber: 8g

- Fat: 12g

Recipe 22: Cucumber Avocado Gazpacho

Ingredients:

- 4 large cucumbers, peeled and chopped

- 2 ripe avocados, peeled and diced

- 1 green bell pepper, diced

- 1/2 red onion, finely chopped

- 2 cloves garlic, minced

- 1/4 cup fresh cilantro, chopped

- Juice of 2 limes

- 3 cups vegetable broth

- Salt and pepper to taste

Instructions:

1. In a blender, combine cucumbers, avocados, bell pepper, red onion, garlic, cilantro, lime juice, and vegetable broth.

2. Blend until smooth.

3. Season with salt and pepper, to taste.

4. Chill in the refrigerator for at least 2 hours before serving.

Nutritional Value (per serving):

- Calories: 220

- Protein: 5g

- Carbohydrates: 25g

- Fiber: 8g

- Fat: 14g

Recipe 23: Walnut and Roasted Red Pepper Hummus

Ingredients:

- 1 can (15 oz) chickpeas, drained and rinsed

- 1/2 cup walnuts

- 1/2 cup roasted red peppers

- 2 cloves garlic

- 3 tablespoons tahini

- Juice of 1 lemon

- 1/4 cup olive oil

- Paprika for garnish

Instructions:

1. In a food processor, blend chickpeas, walnuts, roasted red peppers, garlic, tahini, and lemon juice.

2. While blending, drizzle in olive oil until smooth.

3. Transfer to a serving bowl and sprinkle with paprika.

4. Serve with vegetable sticks or whole-grain crackers.

Nutritional Value (per serving):

- Calories: 260

- Protein: 8g

- Carbohydrates: 15g

- Fiber: 5g

- Fat: 20g

Recipe 24: Quinoa-Stuffed Bell Peppers

Ingredients:

- 4 large bell peppers, halved

- 1 cup quinoa, cooked

- 1 can (15 oz) black beans, drained and rinsed

- 1 cup corn kernels

- 1 cup cherry tomatoes, diced

- 1/4 cup red onion, finely chopped

- 1 teaspoon cumin

- 1/2 teaspoon chili powder

- Juice of 1 lime

- Salt and pepper to taste

Instructions:

1. Preheat the oven to 375°F (190°C).

2. In a bowl, mix cooked quinoa, black beans, corn, cherry tomatoes, red onion, cumin, chili powder, and lime juice.

3. Fill each bell pepper half with the quinoa mixture.

4. Bake for 25–30 minutes until the peppers are tender.

5. Serve with a dollop of guacamole, if desired.

Nutritional Value (per serving):

- Calories: 320

- Protein: 12g

- Carbohydrates: 55g

- Fiber: 12g

- Fat: 5g

Recipe 25: Citrus-marinated Tofu Skewers

Ingredients:

- 1 block extra-firm tofu, cubed

- 1 orange, juiced

- 1 lemon, juiced

- 2 tablespoons soy sauce

- 1 tablespoon maple syrup

- 2 cloves garlic, minced

- 1 teaspoon fresh ginger, grated

- Wooden skewers, soaked in water

Instructions:

1. In a bowl, whisk together orange juice, lemon juice, soy sauce, maple syrup, garlic, and ginger.

2. Marinate tofu cubes in the citrus mixture for at least 30 minutes.

3. Thread marinated tofu onto soaked skewers.

4. Grill or bake until the tofu is golden brown.

5. Serve with a side of quinoa or brown rice.

Nutritional Value (per serving):

- Calories: 280

- Protein: 15g

- Carbohydrates: 25g

- Fiber: 5g

- Fat: 14g

Recipe 26: Mango and Black Bean Quinoa Bowl

Ingredients:

- 1 cup quinoa, cooked

- 1 can (15 oz) black beans, drained and rinsed

- 1 mango, diced

- 1 red bell pepper, diced

- 1/4 cup red onion, finely chopped

- 1/4 cup fresh cilantro, chopped

- Juice of 2 limes

- 2 tablespoons olive oil

- Salt and pepper to taste

Instructions:

1. In a large bowl, combine cooked quinoa, black beans, mango, red bell pepper, red onion, and cilantro.

2. In a small bowl, whisk together the lime juice and olive oil.

3. Pour the dressing over the quinoa mixture and toss until well combined.

4. Season with salt and pepper, to taste.

Nutritional Value (per serving):

- Calories: 340

- Protein: 12g

- Carbohydrates: 55g

- Fiber: 10g

- Fat: 10g

Recipe 27: Coconut-Lime Chia Pudding

Ingredients:

- 1/4 cup chia seeds

- 1 cup coconut milk

- Zest and juice of 1 lime

- 1 tablespoon maple syrup

- Fresh berries for topping

Instructions:

1. In a jar, mix chia seeds, coconut milk, lime zest, lime juice, and maple syrup.

2. Stir well and refrigerate overnight.

3. In the morning, stir the chia pudding to ensure it's well set.

4. Spoon into serving bowls and top with fresh berries.

Nutritional Value (per serving):

- Calories: 180

- Protein: 5g

- Carbohydrates: 15g

- Fiber: 8g

- Fat: 10g

Recipe 28: Stuffed Acorn Squash with Quinoa and Cranberries

Ingredients:

- 2 acorn squash, halved and seeds removed

- 1 cup quinoa, cooked

- 1/2 cup dried cranberries

- 1/4 cup pecans, chopped

- 2 tablespoons maple syrup

- 1 teaspoon cinnamon

- Salt and pepper to taste

Instructions:

1. Preheat the oven to 375°F (190°C).

2. Place acorn squash halves on a baking sheet.

3. In a bowl, mix cooked quinoa, cranberries, pecans, maple syrup, cinnamon, salt, and pepper.

4. Fill each acorn squash half with the quinoa mixture.

5. Bake for 30–40 minutes until the squash is tender.

6. Serve it as a wholesome, autumn-inspired dish.

Nutritional Value (per serving):

- Calories: 320

- Protein: 8g

- Carbohydrates: 60g

- Fiber: 10g

- Fat: 8g

Recipe 29: Blueberry and Almond Overnight Oats

Ingredients:

- 1/2 cup rolled oats

- 1/2 cup almond milk

- 1/4 cup blueberries

- 1 tablespoon almond butter

- 1 teaspoon chia seeds

- 1 teaspoon maple syrup

- Sliced almonds for topping

Instructions:

1. In a jar, combine rolled oats, almond milk, blueberries, almond butter, chia seeds, and maple syrup.

2. Stir well and refrigerate overnight.

3. In the morning, give the oats a good stir and top with sliced almonds before serving.

Nutritional Value (per serving):

- Calories: 280

- Protein: 8g

- Carbohydrates: 35g

- Fiber: 8g

- Fat: 12g

Recipe 30: Sweet Potato and Kale Hash

Ingredients:

- 2 medium sweet potatoes, peeled and grated

- 2 cups kale, stems removed and chopped

- 1 onion, finely chopped

- 2 cloves garlic, minced

- 1 teaspoon smoked paprika

- 1/2 teaspoon cumin

- 2 tablespoons olive oil

- Salt and pepper to taste

Instructions:

1. In a large skillet, heat olive oil over medium heat.

2. Add onion and garlic, and sauté until fragrant.

3. Add grated sweet potatoes, kale, smoked paprika, cumin, salt, and pepper.

4. Cook until sweet potatoes are golden and the kale is wilted.

5. Serve it as a delicious and nutritious breakfast or brunch option.

Nutritional Value (per serving):

- Calories: 260

- Protein: 5g

- Carbohydrates: 35g

- Fiber: 8g

- Fat: 12g

Recipe 31: Pesto Zucchini Noodles with Sun-Dried Tomatoes

Ingredients:

- 4 medium zucchinis, spiralized

- 1 cup fresh basil

- 1/2 cup pine nuts

- 2 cloves garlic

- 1/4 cup nutritional yeast

- Juice of 1 lemon

- 1/3 cup sun-dried tomatoes, chopped

- 3 tablespoons extra-virgin olive oil

- Salt and pepper to taste

Instructions:

1. Spiralize zucchini into noodles.

2. In a food processor, blend basil, pine nuts, garlic, nutritional yeast, and lemon juice.

3. While processing, slowly add olive oil until pesto is well combined.

4. Toss zucchini noodles with pesto and sun-dried tomatoes.

5. Season with salt and pepper before serving.

Nutritional Value (per serving):

- Calories: 290

- Protein: 8g

- Carbohydrates: 20g

- Fiber: 8g

- Fat: 22g

Recipe 32: Turmeric-Ginger Lentil Soup

Ingredients:

- 1 cup dried red lentils

- 1 onion, diced

- 3 carrots, chopped

- 2 celery stalks, sliced

- 2 cloves garlic, minced

- 1 tablespoon fresh ginger, grated

- 1 teaspoon ground turmeric

- 6 cups vegetable broth

- Juice of 1 lemon

- Fresh cilantro for garnish

Instructions:

1. In a pot, sauté onion, carrots, celery, garlic, and ginger until softened.

2. Add lentils, turmeric, and vegetable broth.

3. Simmer for 20-25 minutes until lentils are cooked.

4. Stir in lemon juice.

5. Garnish with fresh cilantro before serving.

Nutritional Value (per serving):

- Calories: 240

- Protein: 15g

- Carbohydrates: 40g

- Fiber: 15g

- Fat: 2g

Recipe 33: Mediterranean Stuffed Pita Pockets

Ingredients:

- 4 whole-grain pita pockets

- 1 cup cooked quinoa

- 1 cup cherry tomatoes, halved

- 1 cucumber, diced

- 1/2 cup Kalamata olives, sliced

- 1/4 cup red onion, finely chopped

- 1/2 cup hummus

- Fresh mint for garnish

Instructions:

1. In a bowl, mix cooked quinoa, cherry tomatoes, cucumber, olives, and red onion.

2. Warm pita pockets in the oven or on a skillet.

3. Spread hummus inside each pita pocket.

4. Stuff with the quinoa mixture.

5. Garnish with fresh mint before serving.

Nutritional Value (per serving):

- Calories: 320

- Protein: 10g

- Carbohydrates: 45g

- Fiber: 10g

- Fat: 12g

Recipe 34: Pineapple and Cilantro Quinoa Salad

Ingredients:

- 1 cup quinoa, cooked and cooled

- 1 cup fresh pineapple, diced

- 1 red bell pepper, diced

- 1/4 cup red onion, finely chopped

- 1/4 cup fresh cilantro, chopped

- Juice of 2 limes

- 2 tablespoons coconut oil

- Salt and pepper to taste

Instructions:

1. In a large bowl, combine quinoa, pineapple, red bell pepper, red onion, and cilantro.

2. In a small bowl, whisk together lime juice and coconut oil.

3. Pour the dressing over the salad and toss until well combined.

4. Season with salt and pepper before serving.

Nutritional Value (per serving):

- Calories: 300

- Protein: 8g

- Carbohydrates: 45g

- Fiber: 7g

- Fat: 10g

Recipe 35: Curry Chickpea and Spinach Stuffed Sweet Potatoes

Ingredients:

- 4 medium sweet potatoes

- 1 can (15 oz) chickpeas, drained and rinsed

- 2 cups fresh spinach

- 1 onion, diced

- 2 cloves garlic, minced

- 1 tablespoon curry powder

- 1/2 teaspoon cumin

- 1/4 cup coconut milk

- Fresh cilantro for garnish

Instructions:

1. Preheat the oven to 400°F (200°C).

2. Bake sweet potatoes until tender, about 45 minutes.

3. In a skillet, sauté onion and garlic until softened.

4. Add chickpeas, spinach, curry powder, and cumin. Cook until spinach wilts.

5. Stir in coconut milk.

6. Slice open sweet potatoes and stuff with the chickpea-spinach mixture.

7. Garnish with fresh cilantro before serving.

Nutritional Value (per serving):

- Calories: 340

- Protein: 10g

- Carbohydrates: 65g

- Fiber: 12g

- Fat: 5g

Recipe 36: Apricot and Almond Quinoa Bowl

Ingredients:

- 1 cup quinoa, cooked

- 1/2 cup dried apricots, chopped

- 1/4 cup almonds, sliced

- 1 tablespoon chia seeds

- 2 tablespoons maple syrup

- 1/2 teaspoon vanilla extract

- Coconut yogurt for serving

Instructions:

1. In a bowl, mix cooked quinoa, dried apricots, almonds, chia seeds, maple syrup, and vanilla extract.

2. Serve in bowls with a dollop of coconut yogurt on top.

Nutritional Value (per serving):

- Calories: 280

- Protein: 7g

- Carbohydrates: 45g

- Fiber: 8g

- Fat: 8g

Recipe 37: Roasted Beet and Walnut Salad

Ingredients:

- 3 medium beets, peeled and diced

- 1/2 cup walnuts, chopped

- 4 cups arugula

- 1/4 cup vegan feta cheese, crumbled

- Balsamic vinaigrette dressing

Instructions:

1. Preheat the oven to 400°F (200°C).

2. Roast diced beets in the oven for 25-30 minutes until tender.

3. In a serving bowl, combine roasted beets, walnuts, arugula, and vegan feta.

4. Drizzle with balsamic vinaigrette before serving.

Nutritional Value (per serving):

- Calories: 280

- Protein: 8g

- Carbohydrates: 30g

- Fiber: 8g

- Fat: 16g

Recipe 38: Spaghetti Squash Primavera

Ingredients:

- 1 medium spaghetti squash

- 1 cup cherry tomatoes, halved

- 1 zucchini, julienned

- 1 carrot, julienned

- 2 cloves garlic, minced

- 1/4 cup fresh basil, chopped

- 2 tablespoons olive oil

- Salt and pepper to taste

Instructions:

1. Preheat the oven to 375°F (190°C).

2. Cut spaghetti squash in half, remove seeds, and roast in the oven for 40-45 minutes.

3. In a skillet, sauté cherry tomatoes, zucchini, carrot, and garlic in olive oil until tender.

4. Scrape the cooked spaghetti squash with a fork to create "noodles."

5. Toss the spaghetti squash with the sautéed vegetables.

6. Garnish with fresh basil and season with salt and pepper.

Nutritional Value (per serving):

- Calories: 250

- Protein: 5g

- Carbohydrates: 30g

- Fiber: 8g

- Fat: 14g

Recipe 39: Cinnamon-Roasted Butternut Squash Soup

Ingredients:

- 1 medium butternut squash, peeled and diced

- 1 onion, diced

- 2 apples, peeled and chopped

- 1 teaspoon cinnamon

- 4 cups vegetable broth

- 1/2 cup coconut milk

- Salt and pepper to taste

- Toasted pumpkin seeds for garnish

Instructions:

1. Preheat the oven to 400°F (200°C).

2. Toss diced butternut squash, onion, and apples with cinnamon.

3. Roast in the oven for 30-35 minutes until vegetables are caramelized.

4. In a pot, combine roasted vegetables, vegetable broth, and coconut milk.

5. Simmer for 15-20 minutes.

6. Blend the soup until smooth.

7. Season with salt and pepper and garnish with toasted pumpkin seeds before serving.

Nutritional Value (per serving):

- Calories: 280

- Protein: 5g

- Carbohydrates: 40g

- Fiber: 10g

- Fat: 12g

Recipe 40: Pistachio-Crusted Baked Cauliflower Steaks

Ingredients:

- 1 large cauliflower head, sliced into steaks

- 1/2 cup shelled pistachios, crushed

- 2 tablespoons Dijon mustard

- 1 tablespoon maple syrup

- 1 tablespoon olive oil

- Salt and pepper to taste

- Lemon wedges for serving

Instructions:

1. Preheat the oven to 400°F (200°C).

2. In a bowl, mix crushed pistachios, Dijon mustard, maple syrup, and olive oil.

3. Brush both sides of the cauliflower steaks with the pistachio mixture.

4. Place on a baking sheet and bake for 25-30 minutes until cauliflower is golden.

5. Serve with lemon wedges.

Nutritional Value (per serving):

- Calories: 220

- Protein: 8g

- Carbohydrates: 20g

- Fiber: 8g

- Fat: 14g

Recipe 41: Raspberry and Mint Chia Seed Lemonade

Ingredients:

- 1/4 cup chia seeds

- 1 cup fresh raspberries

- 1/4 cup fresh mint leaves

- 1/2 cup freshly squeezed lemon juice

- 2 tablespoons agave syrup or honey

- 4 cups water

- Ice cubes for serving

Instructions:

1. In a jar, mix chia seeds and water. Let it sit for 15 minutes until it forms a gel.

2. In a blender, combine raspberries, mint leaves, lemon juice, and agave syrup. Blend until smooth.

3. In a pitcher, combine chia gel and a blended raspberry mixture.

4. Stir well and refrigerate for at least 1 hour.

5. Serve over ice cubes.

Nutritional Value (per serving):

- Calories: 120

- Protein: 3g

- Carbohydrates: 20g

- Fiber: 8g

- Fat: 4g

CONCLUSION

As we savor the last bite of this culinary odyssey through our "Cancer-Fighting Kitchen," let it resonate that every dish is a testament to the healing potential within the realm of plant-based cuisine.

Your journey doesn't conclude with these recipes; rather, it marks the beginning of a lifestyle where the fusion of flavors becomes a formidable ally against disease.

Through the careful selection of ingredients and the artful preparation of each meal, you've not just nourished your body but cultivated a resilience that extends beyond the kitchen.

This cookbook is more than a compilation of recipes; it's an invitation to embrace a philosophy that transcends the plate — a philosophy that values well-being as a sum of conscious choices.

As you relish the tastes and aromas crafted with love and intention, remember that you are sowing the seeds of vitality.

Let this be a catalyst for continued exploration, experimentation, and a joyous commitment to a life where health is not just a goal but a vibrant and enduring reality.

May every bite be a declaration of your commitment to wellness, and may the journey towards a cancer-resistant life be as delightful as the flavors lingering on your palate. Bon appétit and cheers to your health!

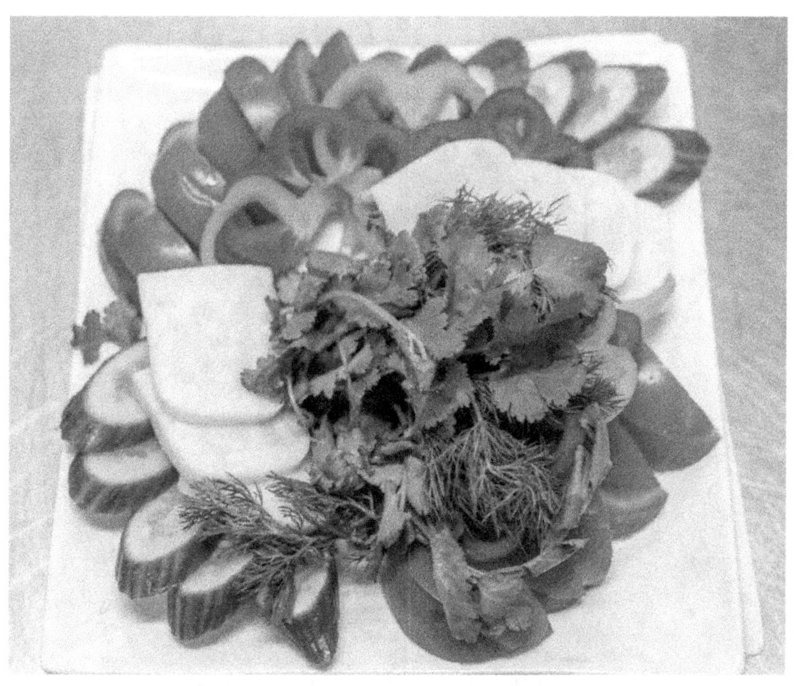